The Secret Solution for Weight Loss Success is…

FORMULA WEIGHT LOSS!!!

by

Lori Martin

THE FIRST STEP

The first step in long-term weight loss success is:

MOTIVATION -- The reason(s) why you want to lose weight.

In the beginning of the weight loss journey, it is necessary for you to write your reason or reasons down. (For some there may be just one motivating reason, and for others there may be many.) Having been a weight loss consultant for many years, I have found that my most successful clients wrote down why they wanted to lose weight, carried this information everywhere they went, and looked at it several times a day. It certainly does help to remind oneself why one is doing something (especially if the task is difficult) because it is so very easy to forget why -- in the moment of temptation -- if one is not constantly reminding oneself of the benefits of staying on track.

The motivation, of course, will vary from person to person. For me, there are many reasons of which I remind myself about when I am tempted to overindulge. The first thing I remind myself about is how "crappy" I felt after the last time I indulged in too much "crap." (Usually the crap involved in these situations is comprised of lots of bad fats -- we're talking the hydrogenated kind -- and too much sugar.) I used to indulge in too many things like sweet rolls and cookies. I would eat one and feel guilty and then punish myself by eating two or three or more (or the whole box or package) instead of just stopping at one. I now make a conscious choice whether I want to indulge in something sweet and allow myself just one serving and I tell myself to slow down and eat it with pleasure instead of with guilt.

I used to have an occasional alcoholic beverage which I rarely ever do now. It's because I discovered that the alcohol just lowers the inhibitions and will in turn make me eat more and drink more. I also discovered that most of them contain sulfites as preservatives (which may not necessarily appear on the label) and this is why my sinuses would get all stuffed up – **NOT FUN!!** (It took me awhile to correlate the two.) So, I decided, who needs the extra empty calories and the stuffy nose? Not to mention the sinus headaches…Not me! I will still have a sip or two of an alcoholic beverage – but only on a special occasion (such as a toast at a wedding). Also, alcohol is very dehydrating. And, when one is dehydrated, one is thirsty. The trouble with being thirsty is that ones body often confuses thirst with hunger. Therefore one is setting oneself up for temptation because of this reason. Who needs that? It's difficult enough to lose weight without indulging in alcohol, so why add it into the mix in the first place?

Besides, all the money saved by not buying a lot of alcohol can go quite far in the way of saving for a trip to a warm climate which can be motivation for staying on track. Who doesn't want to look good in a bathing suit? (Actually through my weight loss consulting I've discovered that there are some people who don't – maybe I'll discuss those reasons later…) Another motivation for me to stay on track and not indulge much in eating another temptation of mine - greasy foods (for me French fries used to be a real killer) was the fact that I discovered that when I overindulged in greasy fried foods, usually the next day my skin would break out in a "lovely" zit -- not to mention two or three! So the next time I'm tempted in the moment with "goodies" I ask myself if I want the zits that come with it. Usually the answer is an adamant "**NO!**" and that is enough to stop me.

I keep reminding myself every day that when I eat better, I feel better and look better 24/7. No longer do I just want to feel better in the moment -- that's no longer good enough for me. I deserve so much better (**I WANT TO FEEL GOOD 24/7!!!**) and so do you! Don't get me wrong. I have not cut anything out from my new way of eating. I have discovered how to have whatever I want ("my cake and eat it too!") and to enjoy eating or drinking without guilt. I call it "mindful eating" versus "mindless eating." There is nothing worse that an "all or nothing" mentality. There is room for imperfection. You just forgive yourself and get right back on track (the next minute -- not the next day) instead of using the "lapse" to overindulge in self-punishment for not being perfect.

SO...go ahead and write down all the reasons why you want to stay on track with this plan, **The Secret Solution For Weight Loss Success is...FORMULA WEIGHT LOSS!!!** The next steps in the plan are soon to follow. Carry your reasons (or reason) with you wherever you go and refer to them often. You will discover (as I did) how much easier it will be to stay on track or to get right back on track immediately this minute – **TODAY!!**

THE SECOND STEP

The second step for weight loss is: **LEARNING HOW TO EAT FOR LONG-LASTING SUCCESS.** You may think that this next step is a bit of a challenge but I'm going to explain it to you simply and then let you figure out your own weight loss plan. You see, I've discovered that most weight loss plans don't work for the rest of your life because they are not personalized and they are not practical. I will share what worked for me. I truly believe it will work for you too. First, you will want to acquire a book or have access to information regarding the calorie content of the food you choose to eat.

Please note: this information needs to provide NOT ONLY the CALORIE content but the FIBER grams and PROTEIN grams of each food item as well.

Now please stay calm. This exercise in education only needs to last a few days or a few weeks -- just until you gain the understanding you need in order to **PERMANENTLY** solve your weight challenges in order to achieve your goal.

Second, you will want to determine your goal weight, because this in turn will allow you to figure out the number of calories you will be able to eat each day in order to not only lose the weight you've determined that you want to lose comfortably, but to be able to learn to eat that same amount in order to **KEEP YOURSELF AT YOUR GOAL WEIGHT FOR THE REST OF YOUR LIFE!!!**

The following is a general formula I use that works well:

For a woman who is five feet tall (all heights are considered without shoes), a weight of 100 pounds is an approximate good weight for her. For each inch over five feet (for example, a medium-framed woman who is five feet seven inches tall) she is allowed five pounds for each of the seven inches she is taller than five feet. Therefore multiply each inch times five. So, for being at least five feet tall, she is allowed 100 pounds and then you add to that 7 x 5 = 35. So, this woman's ideal weight will be 135 (this is the weight she will weigh unclothed first thing in the am before having had anything to eat or drink).

If she is of a small frame, a woman who is 5'7" is still allowed 100 pounds for the being at least five feet tall plus an allowance of three pounds for each of the seven inches she is taller than five feet -- therefore a good weight for her will be 121. If she is of a large frame, multiply the seven inches times an allowance of seven pounds for each inch over 5 feet to come up with an ideal weight of 149.

For a small-framed man, a good general formula will be to use an allowance of five pounds for each inch he is over five feet to come up with an ideal weight of 135 pounds for a man who is 5'7". For a medium-framed man of the same height, a good general formula will be to use an allowance of seven pounds for each inch over five feet to come up with an ideal weight of 149. For a large-framed man, an allowance of ten pounds for each in over five feet will come up with an ideal weight of 170 for a man who is 5'7" tall.

The Secret Solution for Weight Loss Success is ... Formula Weight Loss!!!

I'm hoping by now you're getting the idea of how to figure out your ideal weight. I have a feeling you already intuitively know what that weight is for you and already have a goal in mind.

Now that you have figured out your goal weight, the next step is to figure out the intake of calories that will be your goal number of calories to get used to eating in order to not only **LOSE** the weight but to **MAINTAIN** your ideal weight **FOR THE REST OF YOUR LIFE**!!

The formula that I have found that works best is to use the amount of twelve calories (the number of calories burned each day to maintain each pound of weight on ones body) times the number of pounds you wish to weigh, to arrive at the target number of calories to be consumed each day (without exercise).

If you happen to exercise and enjoy bike riding, for each five miles you ride your bike you will burn approximately 100 calories. Runners or walkers will burn approximately 100 calories for each mile run or walked (walkers burn the same approximate number of calories per mile – it just takes them longer to do it).

So, for example, if a medium-framed 5'5" woman wishes to achieve her ideal goal weight of 125 pounds, in order to figure out the goal number of calories to be consumed each day she will calculate 125 (her goal weight) x 12 (the approximate number of calories it takes to maintain each pound of weight on an inactive body) to equal 1500, the number of calories to be consumed each day for the body to gradually drop to her ideal goal weight of 125 pounds and **STAY THERE!!!** (After all, what is the point of losing weight unless you keep it off?)

Now, if she chooses to regularly walk or run three miles a day, or bikes 15 miles a day, this same woman can consume up to 300 calories more on those days (up from 1500 to 1800 total calories per day!) and still achieve her goal weight and **STAY THERE!!!**. Are you getting the idea?

Now that you understand this concept there are two other things one must do for long-term success:

The **first** is that you include 25 grams of fiber each day (most of us are lucky if we consume 8 or 9 grams) and the **second** is that you consume a minimum of 50 grams of protein each day (preferably at least 20-30 grams of it at breakfast). Most food packaging has this information already written on it.

The Secret Solution for Weight Loss Success is … Formula Weight Loss!!!

What I have found to work best is to jot things down in a notebook and carry it everywhere in order to keep track. You just have one column to write down the food item that you ate, another to write the number of protein grams of that food item, another to write the fiber grams of that food item, and another to write the number of calories contained in that food item. As soon as the total has reached the goal numbers for each category (Protein, Fiber, Calories) for the day (which is at least 50 grams of protein; at least 25 grams of fiber; and, for me, not more than 1620 calories - without exercise) you are finished eating for the day. If you want that 300 calorie dessert, then you must either run or walk 3 miles that day or ride your bike 15 miles. Get the idea? This leads us to the third step...

THE THIRD STEP

The third step in long-term weight loss success is: **GET ACTIVE!!!** There really is no better way to relieve stress. And stress and lack of activity is likely the main reason we overeat in the first place. Think of dogs that get destructive and chew everything in sight. Could it be because they are not getting their daily walks?

I find it to be true for humans too. So find a physical activity that you enjoy doing and research the approximate number of calories burned for that physical activity. You can either add those calories to your base limit of calories to consume for that day, or you can just stick with the base number and get to your goal weight faster!!

SUMMARY

I have just provided all the information you need in order for you to successfully and **PERMANENTLY** achieve your weight loss goal.

Of course, it will take some work and effort on your part.

Everything worthwhile that is ever achieved happens with having a plan and **TAKING ACTION**:

1) Write down your goal and motivations for reaching that goal on a piece of paper. Carry this piece of paper in your purse or pocket everywhere you go referring to it often throughout the day. Tell yourself only positive encouraging things about your ability to achieve your goal, why you want to achieve your goal, and that you are deserving of the success and benefits that come with its achievement. (Please note: this works great with other goals you may have as well!)

2) Keep your food diary (aim for at least five daily servings of fruits and vegetables – this will help you to achieve your goal of 25 grams of fiber each day) until you have learned what it takes to get to and maintain your goal weight.

3) Find an enjoyable activity to do at least three times a week. (Ask yourself if you got in some physical activity yesterday – and if the answer is no – it's time to fit in something today.)

Even if it's just 20 minutes of physical activity – usually you'll burn around 100 extra calories within that period of time. Find a way to break it into two ten minute spurts if that's the only way you can fit it in. The activity in and of itself will already have you feeling so much more relaxed and so much better! Not to mention, it will help get you to your goal faster and help **KEEP YOU THERE...**

CONCLUSION

So there you have it! I have just provided to you all the information it has taken years for me to figure out so that now you too have the knowledge of what it takes to achieve your weight loss goal for life long success.

I truly feel that my method, **The Secret Solution for Weight Loss Success is...FORMULA WEIGHT LOSS!!!,** is the best way to do it.

I wish you all phenomenal health and happiness. I extend my love to all of you who have ever struggled with your weight and hope this information helps you to achieve and maintain your healthy goal weight for the rest of your life.

Lori Martin